making a difference

Caring for Others

Jillian Powell

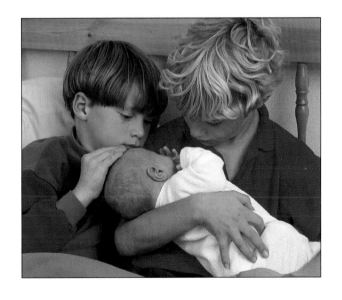

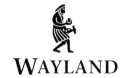

WAYLAND

making a difference

Caring for Others
Caring for the Environment
Caring for Your Pets
Caring for Yourself

Editor: Sarah Doughty
Designer: Jean Wheeler

First published in 1997 by Wayland Publishers Ltd
61 Western Road, Hove, East Sussex BN3 1JD

© Copyright 1997 Wayland Publishers Ltd

British Library Cataloguing in Publication Data
Powell, Jillian
Caring for Others – (Making a Difference series)
1. Caring – Juvenile literature 2. Helping behaviour –
Juvenile literature
I. Title
361

ISBN 0 7502 1943 2

Typeset by Jean Wheeler, in England
Printed and bound by G. Canale & C.S.p.A., Turin

Picture acknowledgements
Chris Fairclough 22 bottom; Eye Ubiquitous 28 top (Tim Hawkins); Impact 12 bottom
(A. Wallerstein), 21 (Bruce Stephens); Life File 13 (John Cox), 27 (David Kampfner);
Reflections 4, 5, 6 both, 7, 10 bottom, 11, 12 top, 16, 17, 24, 26; Robert Harding 9 top, 23;
Sally and Richard Greenhill 10 top, 15; Tony Stone Worldwide 25 (Wayne Eastep), 29
(Myrleen Cate); Wayland Picture Library 9 bottom (Trevor J Hill), 14, 18 (Rupert Horrox,
with special thanks to John Radcliffe Hospital, Oxford), 20 (Rupert Horrox), 22 top (Angus
Blackburn); Zefa 8, 19, 28 bottom. Cover commissioned photography by Angus Blackburn.

Contents

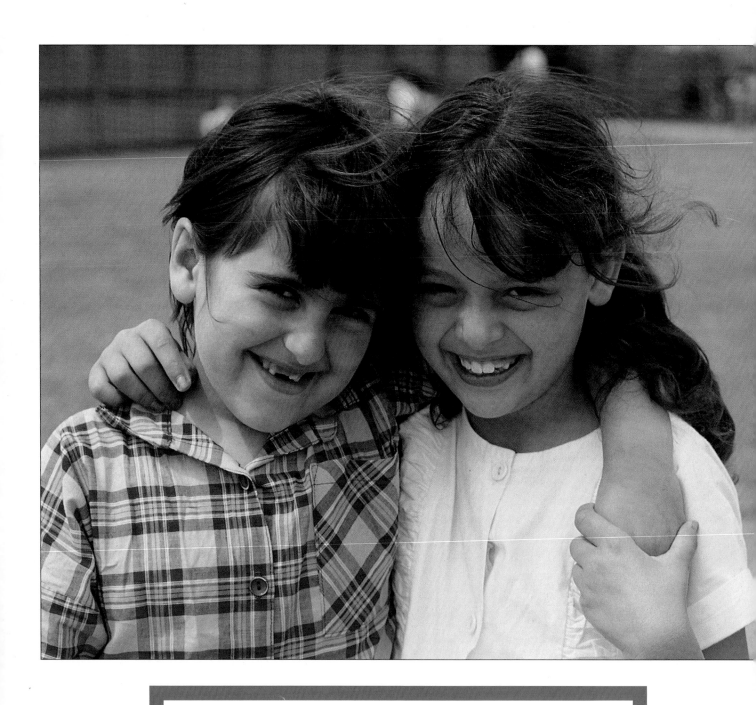

When you care for others,
you think about how they
are feeling.

If they are unhappy, you talk to them to try and help them feel better.

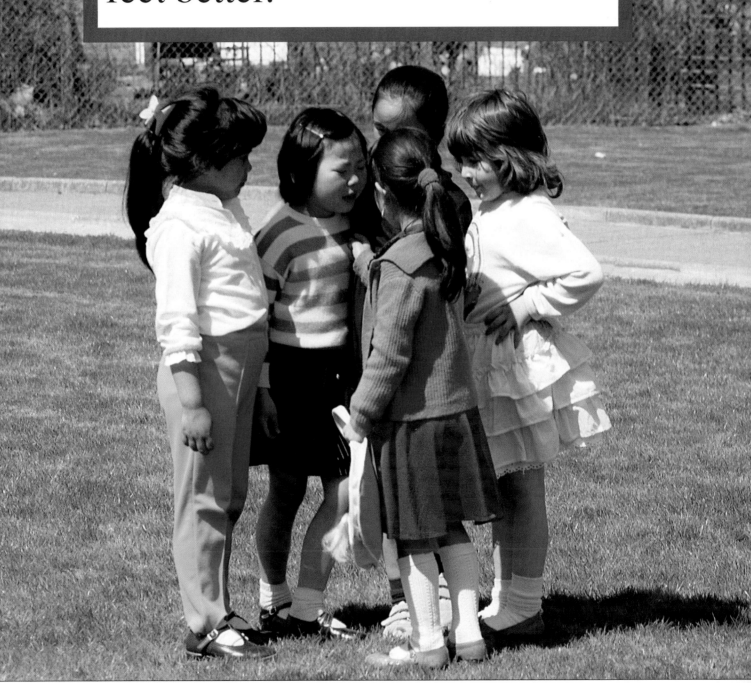

You share happy times too, when you are playing together.

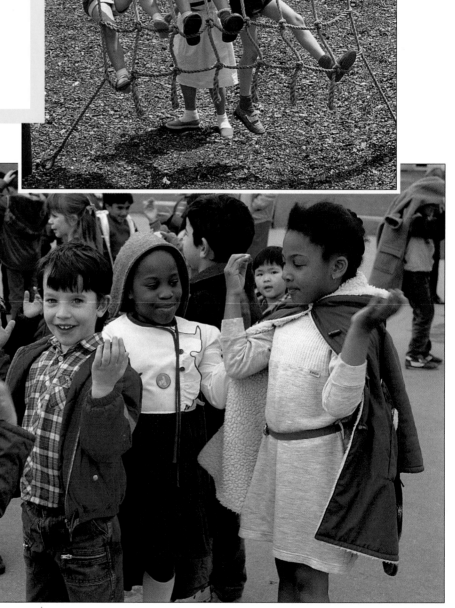

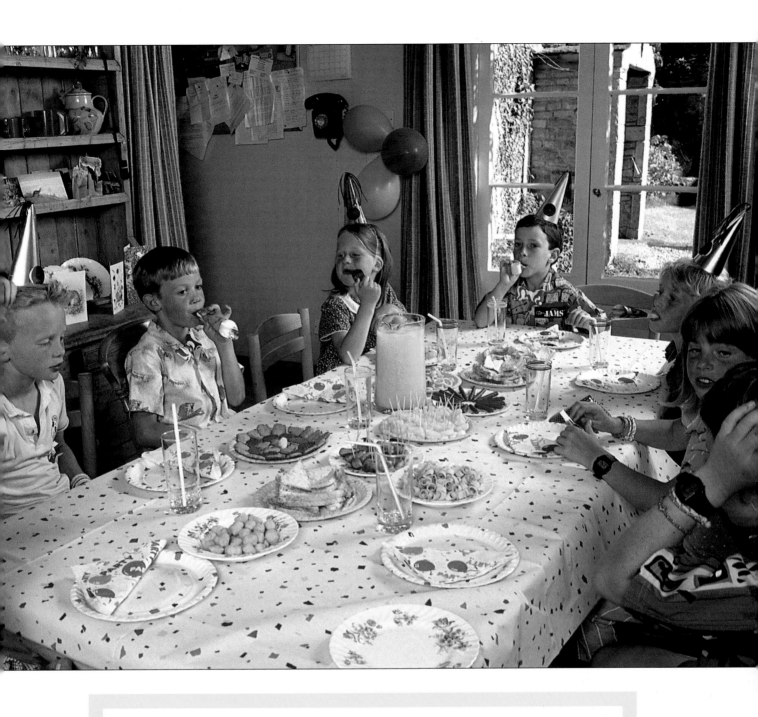

If one of your family or friends
is having a birthday, you help
them have fun.

It is good to share the things you like with your family and friends.

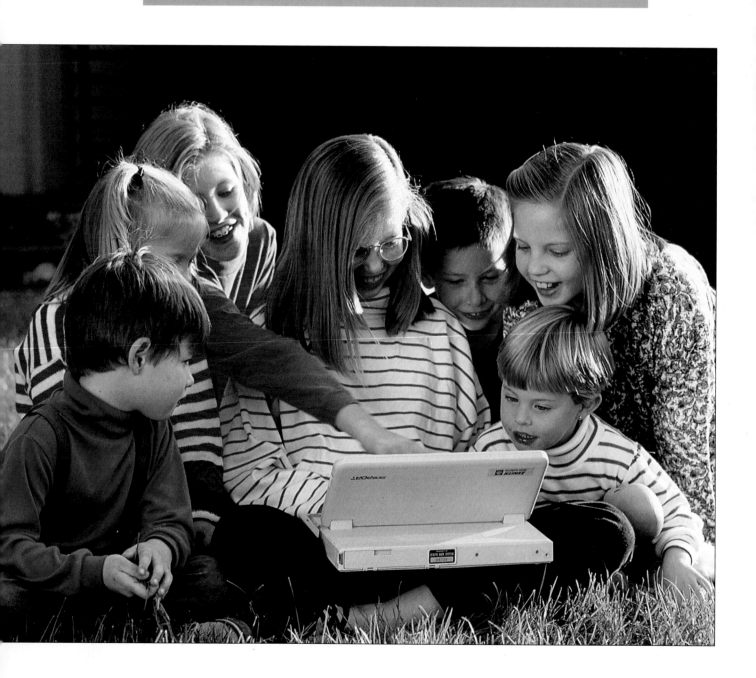

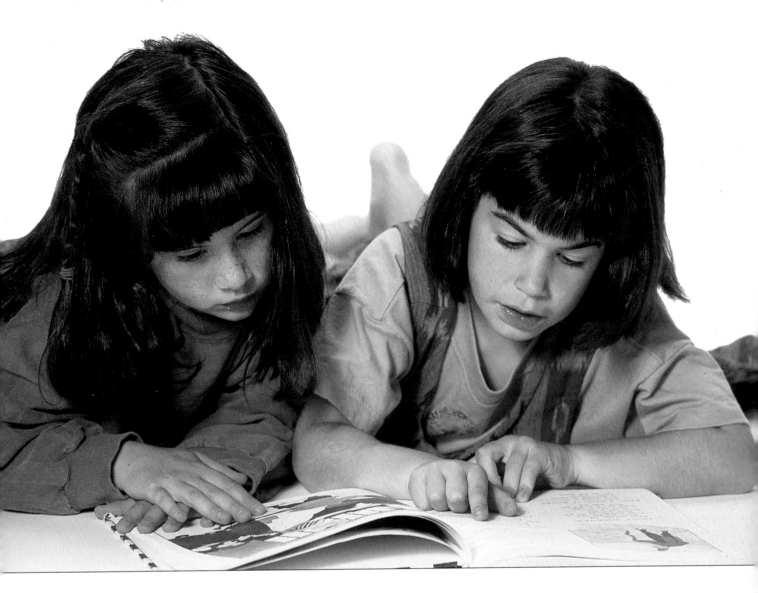

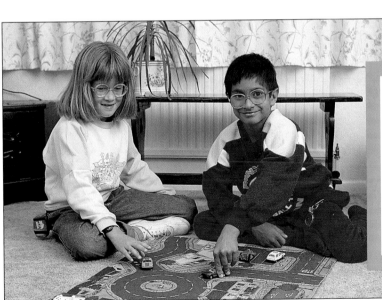

You can play together with your books, toys or games.

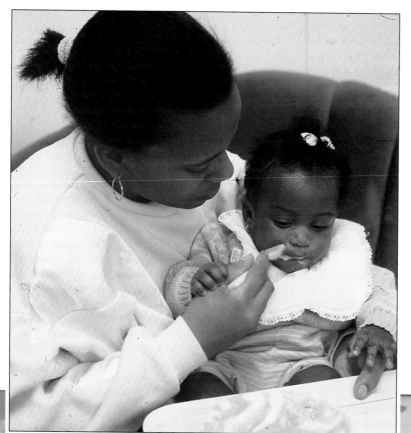

If there is a baby in your family, he or she needs to be cared for all the time.

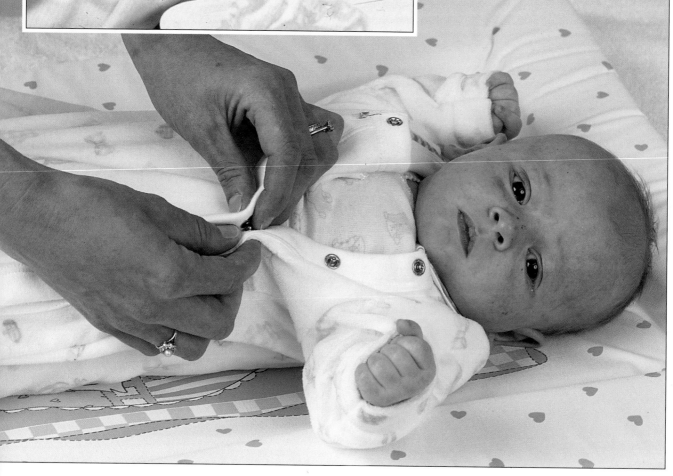

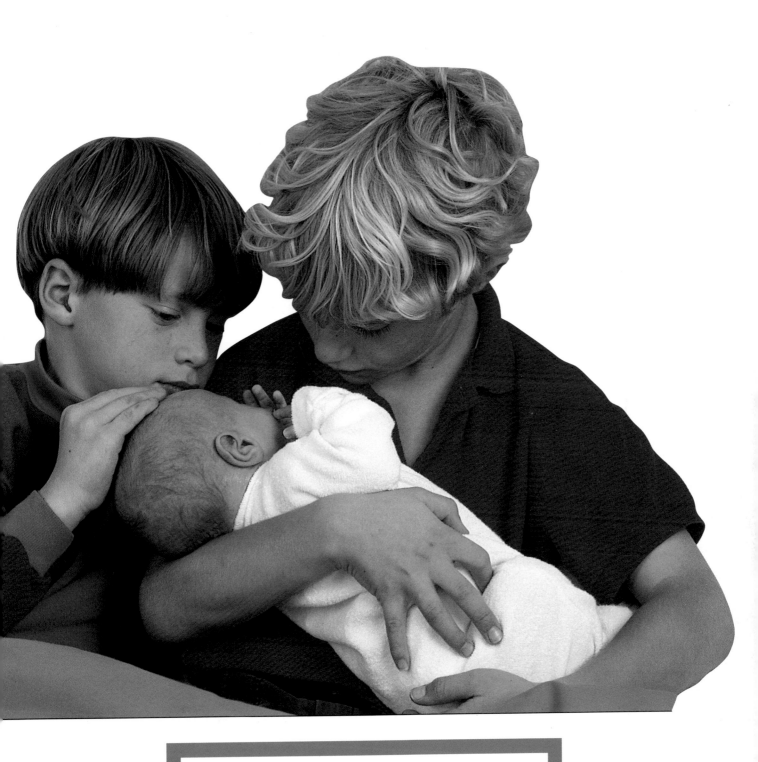

You can help to look after a baby.

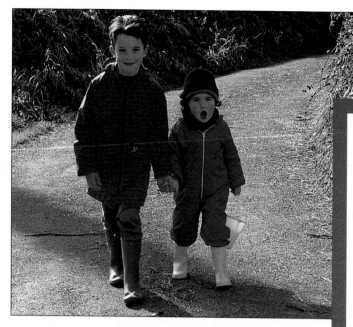

You may have other younger brothers or sisters. You can help to look after them too.

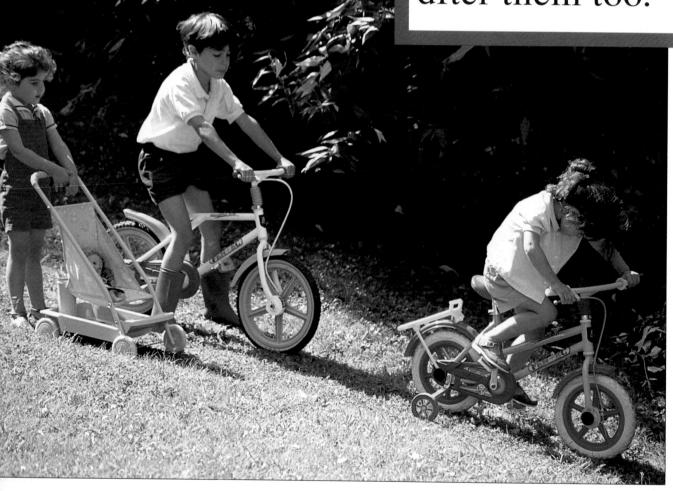

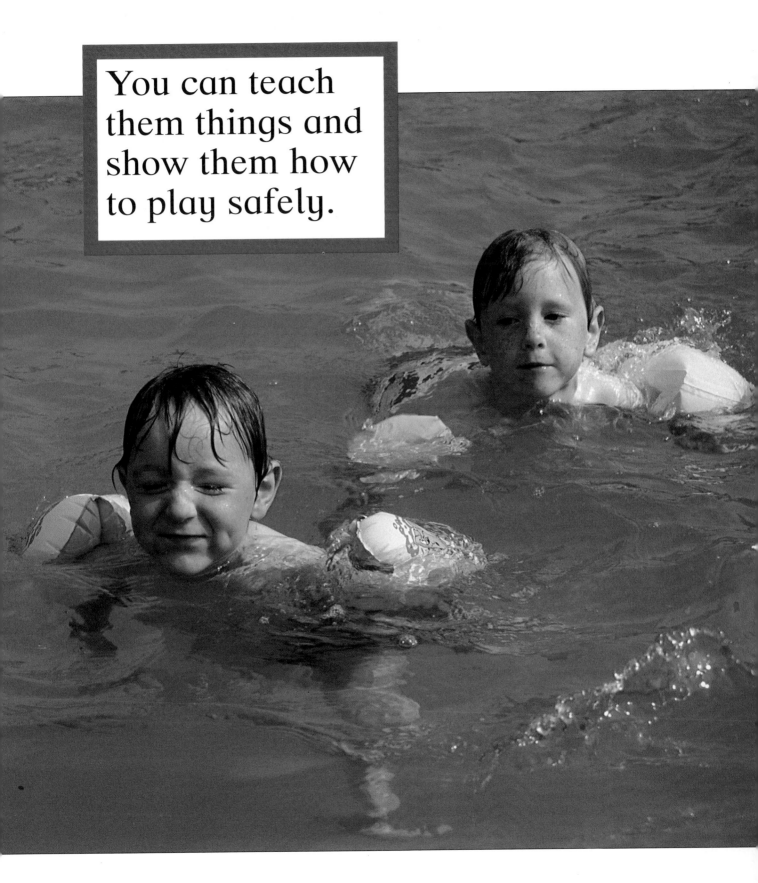

You can teach
them things and
show them how
to play safely.

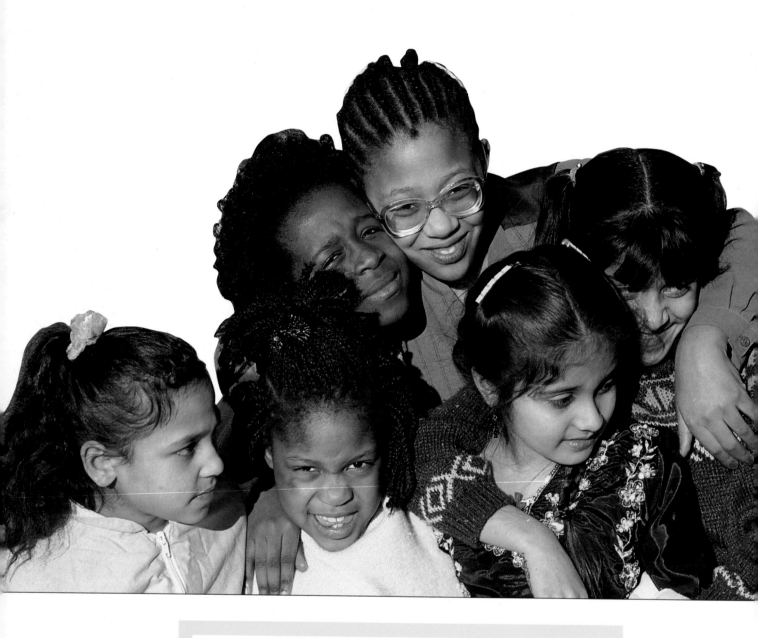

Groups of friends care
for one another. You
may have lots of friends.

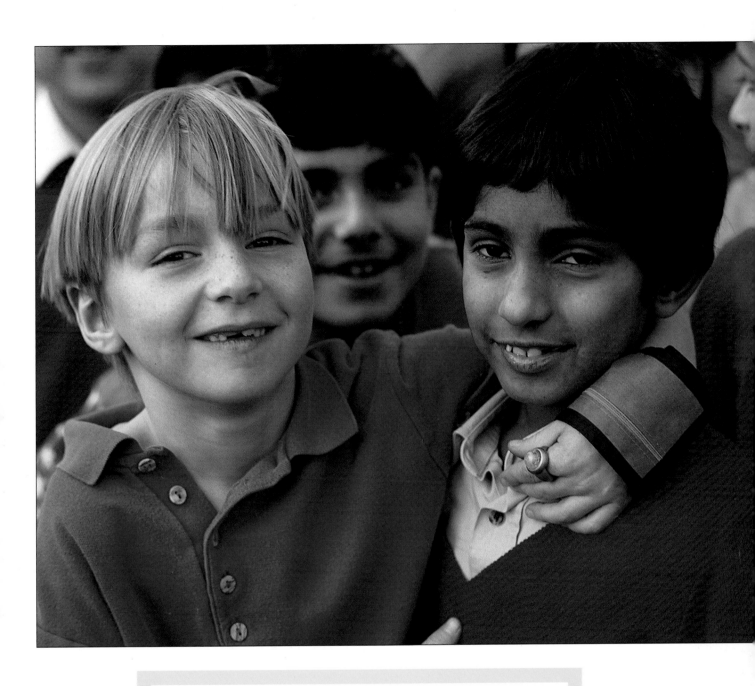

Perhaps you have one
special friend that you
care about the most.

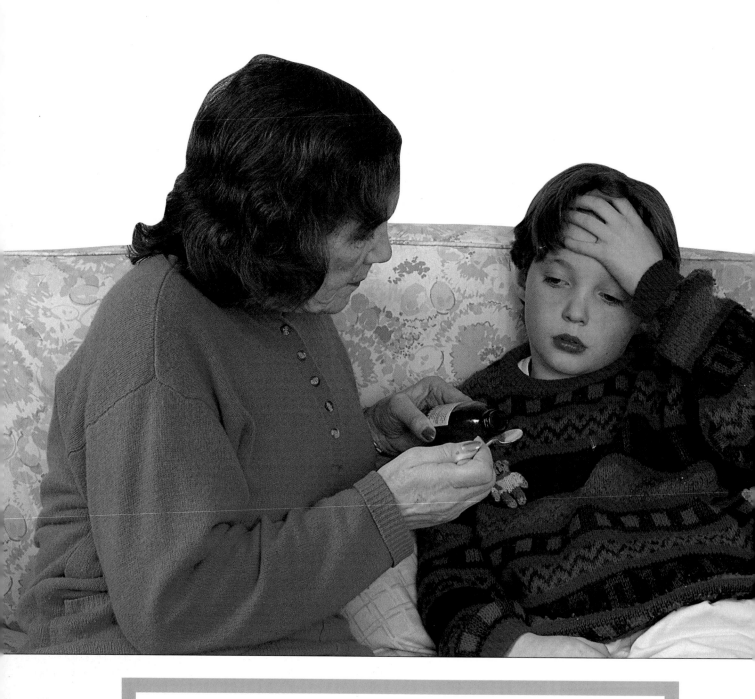

If someone is hurt or sick, they may need special care at home.

You can help by talking to them or playing with them when they begin to feel better.

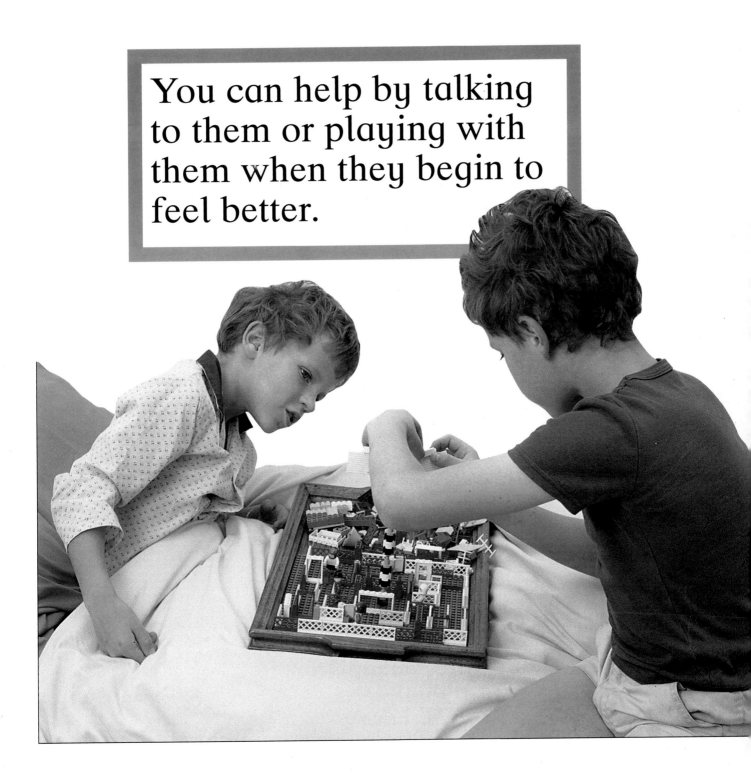

If someone has to go into hospital, they are cared for by nurses and doctors.

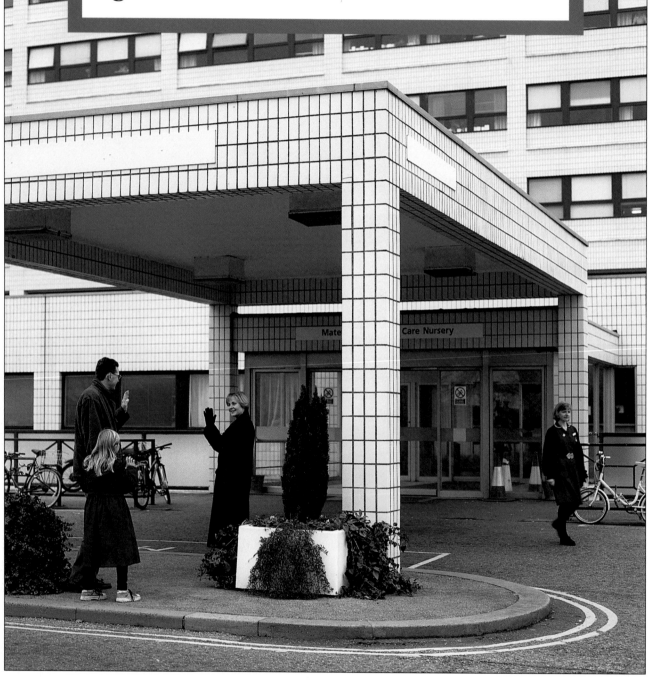

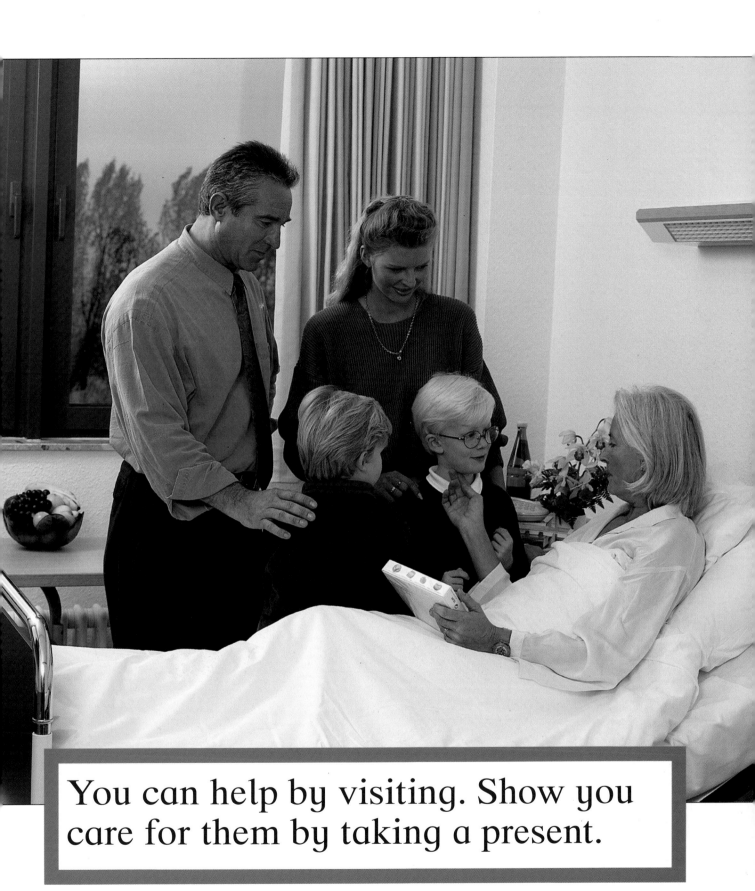

You can help by visiting. Show you care for them by taking a present.

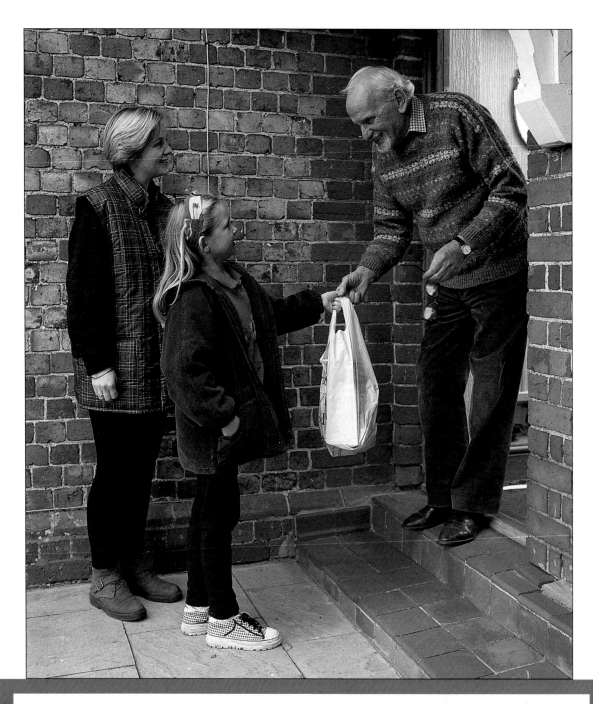

Older people sometimes need help. You can help them by asking if there's anything they need.

They care for you and
give you help in return.

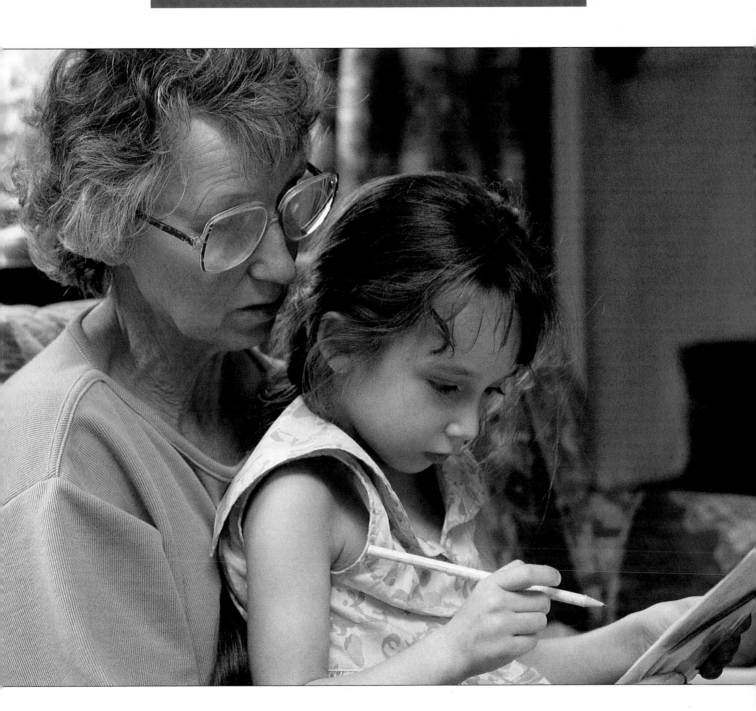

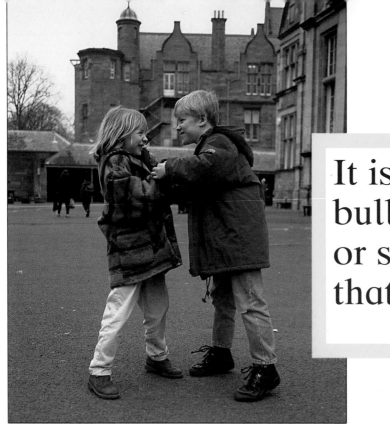

It is wrong to
bully people
or say things
that hurt them.

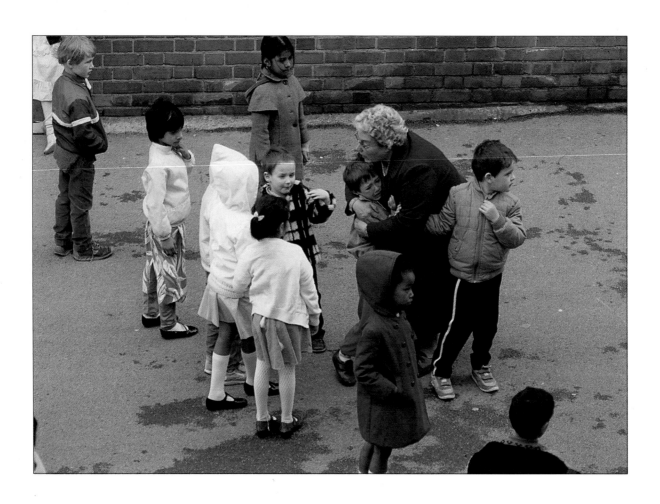

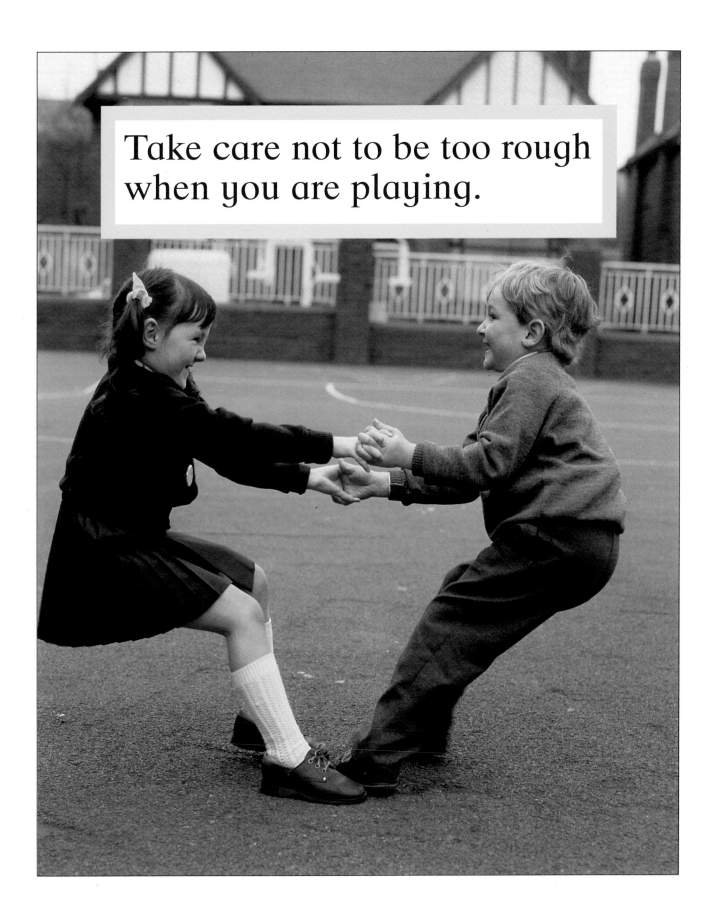

Take care not to be too rough when you are playing.

It is good to tell people that you love and care for them.

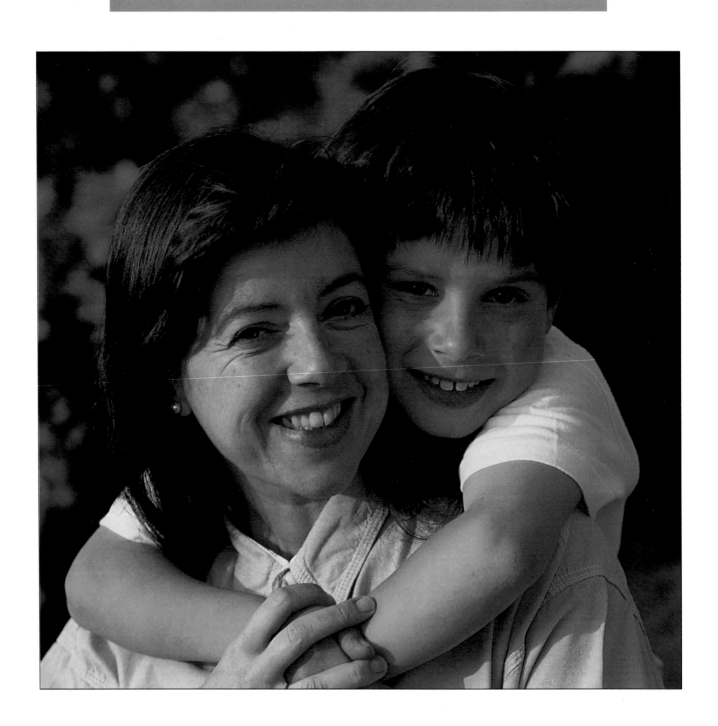

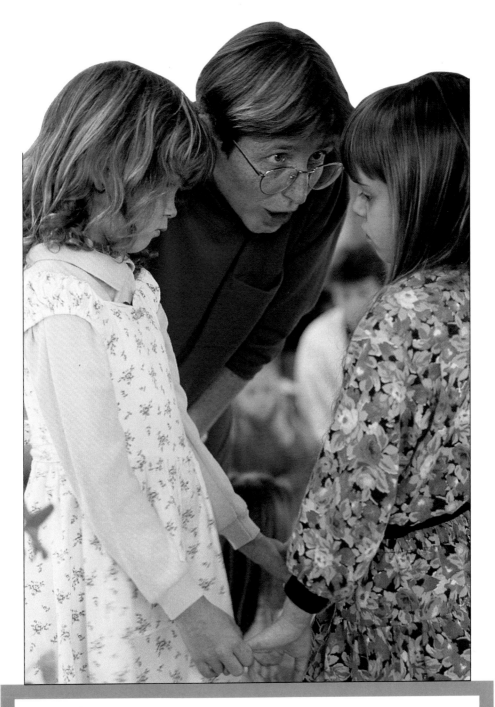

If you have a quarrel with someone, try to make up or you will both feel unhappy.

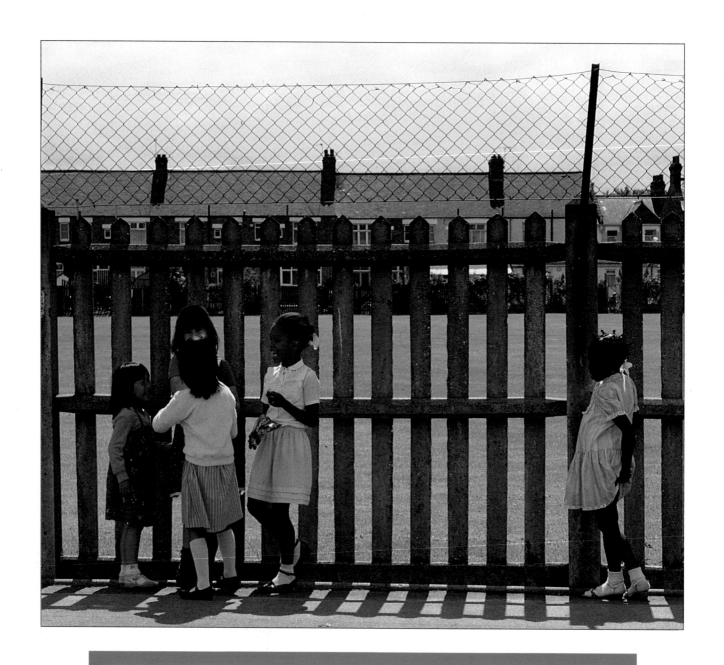

Think about how others are feeling. If someone is new at school, you can help them feel less shy.

You can talk to
them and help them
to join in. You will
soon all be friends.

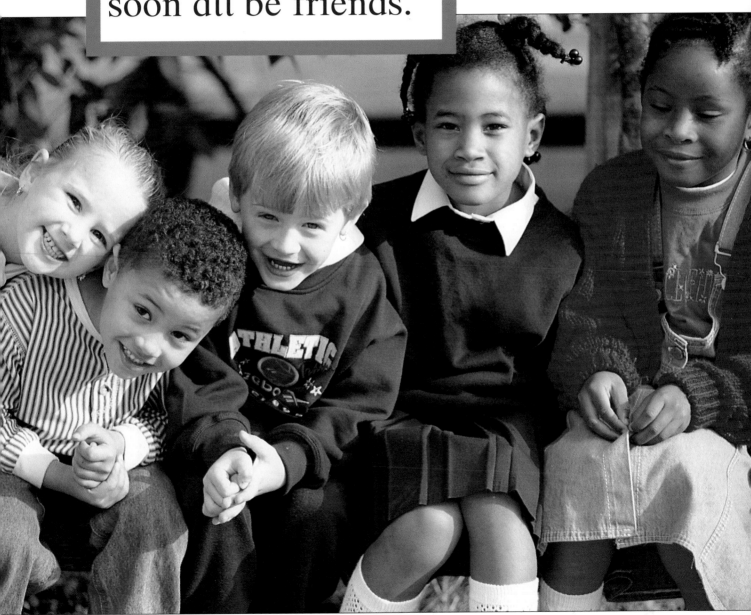

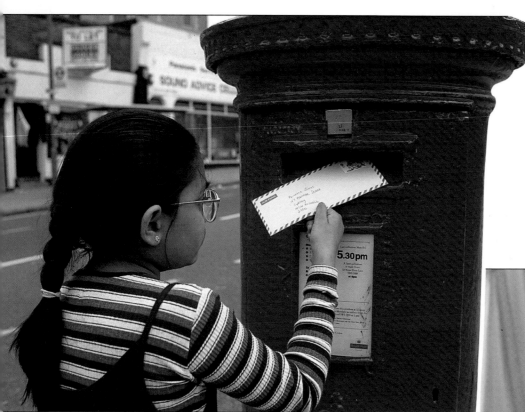

There are lots
of ways to show
people you are
thinking of them.

You can send
them a letter or
make them a card.

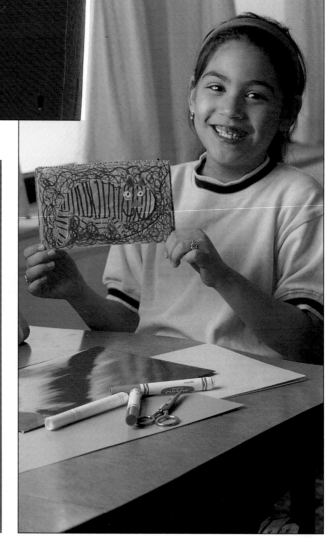

Surprise someone you love with a treat. You can take them breakfast in bed, or give them a present you have made.

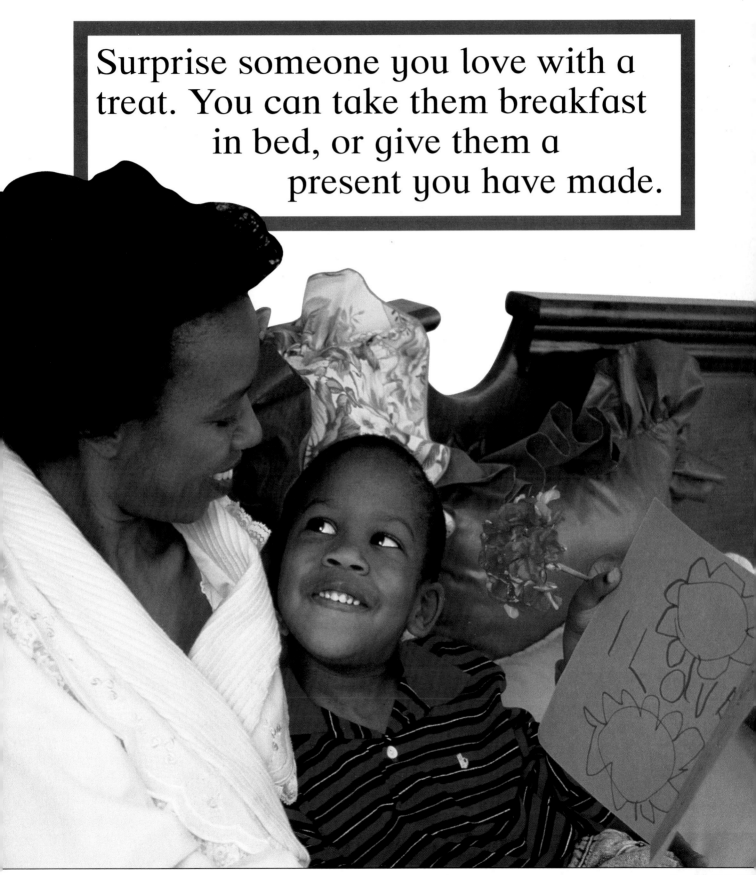

Extension activities

MATHS

Sharing activities: make a real or pretend cake to share into halves, quarters and thirds. Share a bag of sweets or packet of biscuits between larger groups. What do you do if there is a remainder? How many sandwiches can you get from a loaf of bread? And so on.

Play maths games that require turn-taking and sharing. Children can design a game of their own.

ENGLISH

Discuss people who help care for us on a daily basis such as parents, teachers, child-minders. This could develop into a shared writing activity for making a class book.

Make a book about people who care in the community such as doctors, nurses, fire-fighters, etc.

Discuss the effects of language on our feelings, such as kind and cruel words. Make slogans designed to cheer people up.

Write a letter expressing your feelings towards a friend or relative.

MUSIC

Compose happy raps, include caring for others.

Sing, listen to and appreciate the lyrics of caring songs such as 'Robin Hood' or Rolf Harris's 'Horse for two'.

Read hymns and song books looking for lyrics appropriate to the theme of caring for others.

HISTORY

Famous people remembered for their special care towards others: Florence Nightingale, Grace Darling, Robin Hood. When appropriate use biographies.

SCIENCE

Growth and development of human and other animals' babies and their dependence on parent or other adult care. Make time-lines to show the stages and changes from birth to present day of, for example, diet, potty training, pushchairs to walking, and so on (link to History).

Cooking. Make sweets as a surprise present. Discuss the changes made to the ingredients by the effect of combination or heat.

ART AND CRAFT

Design a badge or fridge magnet which expresses a happy slogan. (See English)

Sculpt a clay plaque or model which evokes a caring action.

DESIGN AND TECHNOLOGY

Make cards with a pop-up or sliding mechanism to help cheer someone up.

Display tools such as scissors, bottle opener and tongs. Discuss how they make our life easier. Design a tool that would help someone who cannot bend pick something up from the floor or get something out of the cupboard.

P.E/DANCE/DRAMA

Discuss the merits of, then play: non-competitive games; working in pairs; working as a team.

Explore a range of scenarios which could cause friction, bullying and so on. Through role play how can the children resolve the situation? Discuss sharing, compromise and the action of onlookers.

GEOGRAPHY

Giving directions to the nearest telephone box, health centre or hospital. Following directions, working in pairs one child is led through a simple obstacle course following the verbal directions given by the partner.

Discuss why and how we need to help care for people on a worldwide basis. Use a globe and contact organizations such as Oxfam, Red Cross, Save the Children.

R.E.

Discuss the effects of bullying. Why does it happen? Who does it happen to? Who are the perpetrators? What does it feel like? Explore the actions the children might take.

Sharing the playground. How can those who: want to play football; want peace and quiet and want to play other games share the playground? In small groups design an appropriate use of the playground.

Discuss the story of the Good Samaritan. Discuss the implications of the story on everyday life.

R.E.

- Effects of bullying.
- The story of the Good Samaritan.
- *The Selfish Giant.*
- Sharing the playground.

DESIGN AND TECHNOLOGY

- Display of tools.
- Designing a tool.
- Designing a sweet box.

SCIENCE

- Growth and development.
- The nurture needed by humans and animals.
- Cooking.

ENGLISH

- Discussion of people who care for us.
- Discussion of the effects of language on our feelings.
- Bookmaking.
- Shared writing.
- Letter writing.

HISTORY

- Famous careers in history.

Caring for others
Topic web

MUSIC

- Composing raps.
- Singing.
- Exploring lyrics.

GEOGRAPHY

- Giving and following instructions.
- Discussing aid world wide.

MATHS

- Sharing activities.
- Turn-taking activities.

ART AND CRAFT

- Designing a badge for a fridge magnet.
- Sculpting a clay plaque.

P.E./DANCE/DRAMA

- Non-competitive games.
- Working in pairs.
- Role playing.
- Team work.

Glossary

bully To make someone upset or afraid.

quarrel When people get cross with each other and have a row.

special Very important.

treat Something special to enjoy.

Books to read

How do I feel about...Bullies and Gangs by Julie Johnson (Franklin Watts, 1996)

How do I feel about...Loneliness and Making Friends by Julie Johnson (Franklin Watts, 1996)

Who are Your Family? by Jillian Powell (Wayland, 1993)

Who are Your Friends? by Jillian Powell (Wayland, 1993)

Index